HEALTH BENEFITS
OF SEX
DURING PREGNANCY.

By

Sommy Mirrian.

Table Of Content

CHAPTER ONE

INTRODUCTION TO DIBERS HEALTH BENEFITS DURING PREGNANCY.

It is safe to have sex during pregnancy unless a doctor or midwife advised otherwise.

Infact sex urge or drive may increase at certain stages of pregnancy as a result of increase in various hormones.

The hormones responsible for high sex drive or urge are ESTROGEN, PROGESTERONE, and TESTOSTERONE.

Talking openly about sex can help both partners to enjoy every bit of sex throughout the journey of pregnancy.

Sex during pregnancy prepares pregnant women for child birth.

It prepares the pelvic muscles and cervix for birth. Sex during pregnancy helps increase oxytocin levels, and it is often suggested to pregnant women, particularly those who have already reached the ninth-month mark.

CHAPTER TWO

WHAT IS SEXUAL INTERCOURSE?

Sexual intercourse also known as Coitus or Copulation, is a sexual activity involving the insertion and thrusting of the penis inside the vagina for sexual pleasure, reproduction or even for both.

Sex may be divided into 3 main categories:

1. Vaginal
2. Anal
3. Oral

1. Vaginal sex(Penis -in-vagina intercourse)
2. Oral sex(Mouth -to-genital contact)
3. Anal sex(Penis-in-butt intercourse)

Others may include; Fingering or hand jobs(Hand-to-genital contact).

A 7-STEPS GUIDE TO HAVE AN AMAZING SEX

- Make sure your partner wants to have sex.
- When your partner agrees, pick a comfortable table spot.
- Kiss and caress your partner (foreplay).
- Initiate sex when the moment is right.
- Increase the process of love-making
- Wait for the climax
- Then attain your orgasm.

CHAPTER THREE

PREGNANCY.

Pregnancy is the time during one or more offspring develops inside a woman's uterus or womb.

Pregnancy usually lasts about 40 weeks, or just over 9 months, as measured from last menstrual period to delivery.

Pregnancy is roughly divided into 3 stages know as TRIMESTERS of about 3 months each.

1. **FIRST TRIMESTER:**

This is from conception period to 12 weeks of pregnancy. (1-3months).

2. **SECOND TRIMESTER:**
This from 13 weeks to 27 weeks of pregnancy (3-6months).

3. **THIRD TRIMESTER:**
This from 28 weeks to 40 weeks of pregnancy (6_9months).

There are many symptoms of pregnancy but early symptoms an individual may experience includes, missed period, nausea and vomiting, frequent urination, early morning sickness, breast tenderness, fatigue, backache and food cravings.

NOTE: It is possible for an individual to still see her period while pregnant till the end of her first trimester.

Some women may begin noticing the first early signs and symptoms of pregnancy a week or two weeks after conception, while others will start to feel symptoms closer to four or five weeks after conception.

Some women may not feel symptoms until farther into pregnancy.

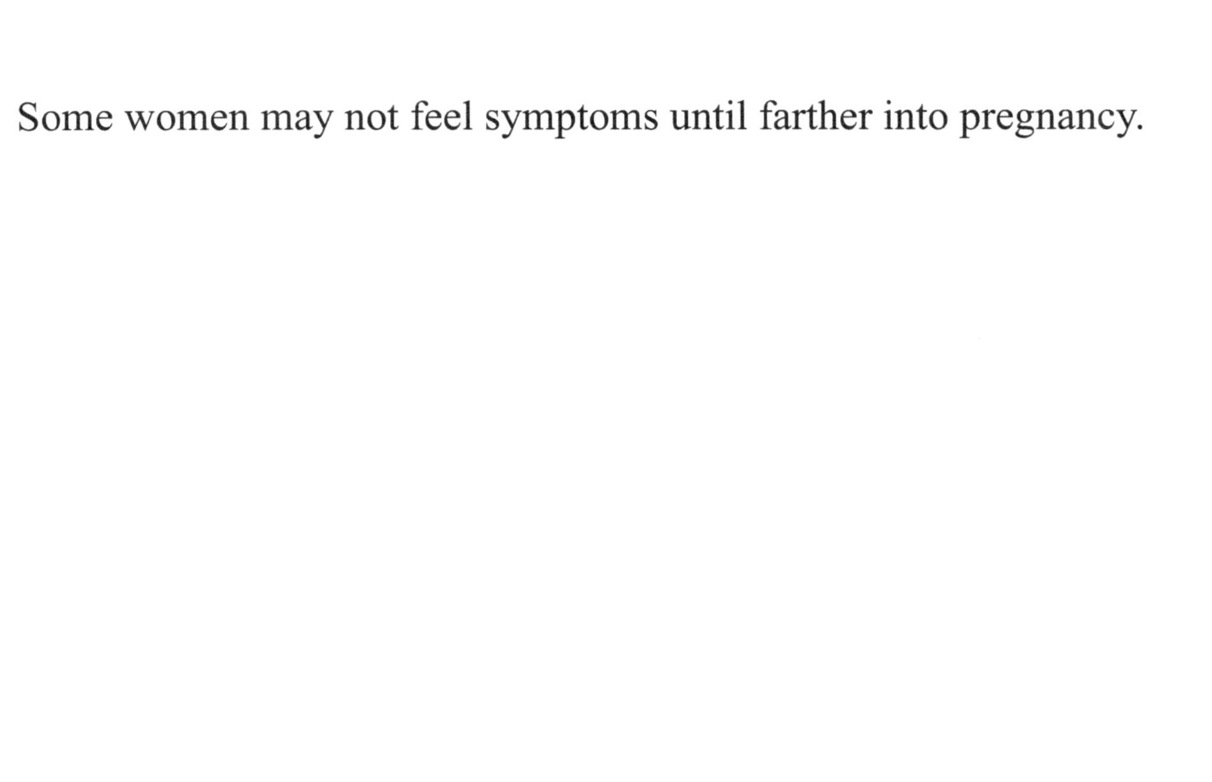

DANGER SIGNS IN PREGNANCY ESPECIALLY IN FIRST TRIMESTER

Vaginal bleeding or spotting: This indicate a miscarriage and is a serious condition that requires immediate medical attention.

Vaginal discharge: This means a vaginal discharge with a bad or foul smell, which is usually as a result of infection, which can be very dangerous to the pregnancy and therefore requires a medical attention.

Blurred vision and Dizziness: This usually a sign of pre-eclampsia and low blood pressure which can be very dangerous during pregnancy and must be addressed with immediate effect.

Severe and persistent high fever: This some times can as well be a sign of infection, which is unsafe to the pregnancy mother.

Severe abdominal pains or cramps: This can be a sign of a threatening abortion and therefore must be addressed immediately by a doctor.

Consistent ANTENATAL CARE is very essential during pregnancy and as well will help to keep the mother and the child very safe, and mostly aid to safe delivery of the baby and sound health to both mother and her child.

Good health education on safe act during pregnancy will as well keep the pregnant mother in-check with her lifestyle during the journey of pregnancy.

CHAPTER FOUR

EFFECT OF PREGNANCY ON SEX URGE OR DRIVE.

It is common for sex drive to be higher or lower than before during pregnancy.

This can be because of changes in the body, hormones, mood, and energy levels. These changes that occurs during this period are very natural and doesn't cause for alarm.

A boost of hormones and increased blood flow to the genitals increase a person's sex urge, particularly in second trimester.

Other people may experience a decrease in their sex drive which is caused by fluctuating hormones, there by feeling less comfortable in their body and decreased in energy level.

Pregnancy can as well affect the sex urge of a pregnant partner.

Some people may experience an increase attraction to their pregnant partner due to the changes in their body shape and increase in their breast size.

Never the less, it is very essential to be open about sex to make sure both partners are comfortable and as well satisfied with their sexual life.

CHAPTER FIVE

DIFFERENT SEX POSITIONS.

When it comes to sex positions, one might have few favorites that he or she rely on.

Sex positions helps to increase comfort during sexual intercourse.

This sex positions helps in lasting longer and as well more fun in the bedroom. Sex positions also helps one reach his or her orgasm too quickly during sexual intercourse.

There are wide range of sex positions but will discuss few below;

COWGIRL: In this sex position, the man is meant to lie on his back, while he allows his partner to mount on him, the woman straddle her hips, and the man will insert his penis from an upright position.

Then the lady can then ride the penis like a cowgirl riding a bull.

In this sex position the woman has almost complete control of the penetration.

Most ladies love this sex position because it puts her in control of the sex session.

SPOONING POSITION: In this position both partners lies on their sides, the man front pressing against the woman back like spooning cuddle position.

The woman should separate her legs a little, find her vagina with your hand and insert your penis from behind.

The short strokes target her G-spot, making it a great one for her. Focus on grinding your hips against her butt, and consider stimulating her clitoris with your fingers.

This sex position can help you bring her to her orgasm and make her feel very good.

In this sex position the man is the the big spoon and the woman is the small spoon.

 SIDE BY SIDE POSITION: This sex position is similar to spoon position, but in this particular position the both partners faces each other.

Both partners lying side face to face, the woman lifts her free leg and wraps it around the partner's hip, there by giving him access to her vagina for penetration.

In this sex position both partners can control how deep they thrust. This sex position is both active and passive for both partners.

YAB-YUM POSITION: In this sex position the man sits on the the bed or the floor, and the woman straddles his hip, facing him and allowing him to penetrate her from front.

In this position the man can't thrust indiscriminately while holding himself up a his partner. This sex position is a very intimate position great for pleasing your partner and getting feedback from her reactions.

CROSS POSITION: This sex position involves the man lying on his side and the woman on her back, her torso at 90 degree angle to your torso, her legs draped over your pelvis.

Thrust her and penetrate into her thighs.

In this sex position there is not much range of motion for the man to go nuts, nor easy to thrust uncontrollably.

MISSIONARY POSITION: This sex position is the easiest position. In this sex position the man is the one doing all the thrusting and he has access to deep penetration.

This position required the man to thrust his penis deep and leave it there, grinding his hips against her.

It is easier to keep penis from being overstimulated.

Meanwhile, the woman the front action grinding.

This is because it rubs her clitoris while filling her vagina fully.

SIT ON THE THRONE: In this sex position, the man is to sit on a chair and have the woman stand with her back facing him, then lower into a seated position on his lap, inserting his penis as she does so.

 In this sex position the woman has more control and usually grind against the man hips, enjoying the deep penetration without long or fast thrust.

DOGGY STYLE POSITION: In this sex position, the woman bends over, crouched on all fours (usually on hands and knees), allow the man to penetrate from back.

This sex position basically comfortable for men and as well can make them ejaculate quick.

CHAPTER SIX

BEST SEX POSITIONS DURING PREGNANCY.

Sex is something that can happen throughout the pregnancy, until the moment of delivery.

Though at times, sex during pregnancy might feel uncomfortable due to changes in hormones lower sex drive or age and a growing belly.

But practicing different sex position can reduce discomfort and help a partner have sex around the growing belly.

Below are four different sex positions that are safe to try while pregnant.

1. STANDING SEX FROM BEHIND:

 The best time to try this, is in the first and second trimester.
Stand on the ground while facing a wall, place your hand against the wall and lean in slightly for added stability.

Have your partner enter you from behind holding your hips for added support.

2. SEX FROM BEHIND:

When to try it, first second and third trimester.
Kneel on the bed why putting your hands against the wall for support.

During the first trimester, when the belly is not yet heavy, you could also get all fours and allow your partner enter you from behind.

3. PREGNANT PERSON ON TOP:

This can be done both in first, second, and third trimester. Your partner lies on his back with his knees straight or bent.

 Straddle your partner, facing him and bending your knees, so he can penetrate you.

Either you or your partner can stimulate your clitoris from this position.

 Optional: lean back to take extra weight off your belly and widen your leg stance for deeper penetration.

For more shallow penetration, narrow your leg stance or lean forward.

4. **DOGGY STYLE:**

This can be done in first, second and third trimester.

The pregnant woman bends over, crouches on all fours (hands and knees), while the partner enter from the back.

5. **REVERSE COWGIRL:**

This position can be practice both in first, second, and third trimester.

The man lies on his back with his knees straight or bent. Straddle your partner, facing away from him, so he can penetrate you.

The partner may be able to stimulate your clitoris, and you may also able to stimulate your clitoris yourself.

NOTE: laying on your back during sex after 20 weeks (5months) can compress your VENA CAVA, the major blood vessels which helps with circulation through your body and to your baby.

During the later stage of pregnancy, the couple should not choose positions that will put pressure on the pregnant belly.

Examples MISSIONARY POSITION this is because if the woman lies on her back, the weight of the baby will put extra pressure on her internal organs or major arteries.

Most times a pregnant woman feel more comfortable in a position where she can control the depth and speed of penetration.

CHAPTER SEVEN

HEALTH BENEFITS OF SEX

Sex is superb beneficial to our health.

Sex activates a variety of neurotransmitters that impact not only on the hormones but on several other organs in the bodies.

Though sex isn't enough exercise, but it can as well be considered as a light exercise.

Some research has proved that menwho had more frequent penile-vagina intercourse (PVI) is less prone of developing prostate cancer.

Sex increases the flow of blood to the vagina, reducing vaginal ATROPHY.

Sex improve cardiovascular health and helps to keep the immune system in check and as well in betterment of the immune system.

Sexual intercourse helps to lower blood pressure, help releases good hormones like ENDORPHINS.

The act of sexual intercourse can help strengthen pelvic floor of a woman.

A improvesstrengthen pelvic floor also offer benefits like less pain during sexual intercourse and it also helps reduced the chance of a vaginal prolapse.

Sexual activity in women bladder control, reduce incontinence.

 Sex helps to improve fertility in women, build stronger pelvic muscles, helps produce more vaginal lubrication and most help protect against ENDOMETRIOSIS, or the growing of tissue outside the uterus.

Sex has a benefits on mental health, this is because sexual activity, with a partner can increased the level of trust, intimacy, and love in a relationship.

It increased satisfaction with a mental health.

Sex can reduce stress and anxiety and as well increased happiness. Sexual intercourse improved the ability to perceive, identify and express emotions.

Sex can increase feeling of desire and improve libido.

CHAPTER EIGHT

HEALTH BENEFITS OF SEX DURING PREGNANCY

Sex during pregnancy prepares the woman for childbirth.

More over, vaginal intercourse is very advantageous because it prepares the pelvic muscles and cervix for childbirth.

Sex during pregnancy helps increase OXYTOCIN levels, and it is often suggested to pregnant women, particularly those who have already reached the ninth -month mark.

Sex during pregnancy is good for both mother and the baby.

Good sexual intercourse can help the woman sleep better, lower her blood pressure and most likely to even make her more happier.

When a pregnant woman reaches an orgasm during sexual intercourse, the body releases the hormone OXYTOCIN, which can promote pain relief and increase feeling of intimacy between the woman and her partner.

When a pregnant woman near her due date, orgasm during sexual intercourse helps to put the woman into labor more quickly.

This is because the uterus contracts when the woman reaches her orgasm.

NOTE: This won't cause the woman to go into premature labor.

Sexual activity during pregnancy aids in vaginal lubrication.

Sexual intercourse during pregnancy tends to increase bonding between partners.

Sex during pregnancy increases orgasm which releases endorphins that help the mother and the baby happy and relaxed.

IMPORTANT: Allowing your husband to suck your breast during pregnancy helps the nipples to be out and make it very easier for the baby to latch on after delivery.

Sucking the breast during pregnancy also prepares the mother's mind for breastfeeding.

It is also wonderful to gently press and touch your breasts during pregnancy.

During pregnancy the developing baby is protected by the amiotic fluid in the uterus, and of course strong muscles of the uterus.

Therefore, sexual activity won't affect the baby, as long as the mother has no complications such as PRETERM LABOR and PLACENTA PROBLEM.

Provided the mother is having a normal and uncomplicated pregnancy, she can continue to have sex right up until her water breaks or she goes into labor.

CHAPTER NINE

WHEN TO AVOID SEX DURING PREGNANCY.

Spotting or mild cramps can happen after sex when pregnant, but if the cramps or spotting doesn't stopped few minutes after the sex, then the Doctor's or a Healthcare provider should be called.

Sex should totally be discontinue when there is heavy bleeding in pregnancy.

SEXUAL INTERCOURSE SHOULD BE STRICKLY AVOID DURING PREGNANCY IF THE WOMAN HAS EXPERIENCE THE FOLLOWING:

Problems with the cervix because this could increase the possibility of miscarriage or going into early labor.

Placenta previa, this is where the placenta partially or entirely covers the entrance of the cervix.

Cervical incompetence, this is where the cervix opens prematurely. Water broken, which may increase the risk of infection when practicing sex.

SEXUAL BEHAVIOR TO AVOID DURING PREGNANCY.

Any pregnant woman must not allow her partner to blow air into the vaginal region.

Blowing air into the vagina can cause an sir embolism, and this can be potentially serious for the mother and as well the baby.

Pregnant woman should not have sex with partner who have sexually transmitted diseases, as there are great chances of being infected with sexually transmitted like Hiv.

The disease can easily be transmitted to the baby, if the woman have unprotected sexual intercourse with such partner.

A pregnant woman experiencing frequent abdominal pains, must also avoid sex during her period of pregnancy .

CHAPTER TEN.

DOES SEX TRIGGER LABOR?

Many studies have concluded that vaginal sex during pregnancy has no links in an increased risk of preterm labor or premature birth.

However, if a doctor considers someone to be at high risk, the doctor may recommend that the person avoids sexual intercourse during her period of pregnancy or in her later stages of pregnancy.

It is possible that an orgasm or sexual penetration could induce:

BRAXTON HICKS contractions late in pregnancy.

BRAXTON HICKS are mild contractions that some women experience towards the end of their pregnancy.

However, these contractions doesn't induce labor and so should not be a cause for concern.

Having an orgasm leads to contractions of the uterus, and it can be quite powerful and last up to half an hour.

But it is not to potentially help to initiate or induce labor.

Health Benefits of sex During Pregnancy.